Lizandra Espinosa Carás
Mirtha María Peláez Vega

THE CAGUT

Lizandra Espinosa Carás
Mirtha María Peláez Vega

THE CAGUT

Results of its implementation in patients with chronic pelvic inflammatory disease.

ScienciaScripts

Imprint

Any brand names and product names mentioned in this book are subject to trademark, brand or patent protection and are trademarks or registered trademarks of their respective holders. The use of brand names, product names, common names, trade names, product descriptions etc. even without a particular marking in this work is in no way to be construed to mean that such names may be regarded as unrestricted in respect of trademark and brand protection legislation and could thus be used by anyone.

Cover image: www.ingimage.com

This book is a translation from the original published under ISBN 978-613-9-09261-1.

Publisher:
Sciencia Scripts
is a trademark of
Dodo Books Indian Ocean Ltd. and OmniScriptum S.R.L publishing group

120 High Road, East Finchley, London, N2 9ED, United Kingdom
Str. Armeneasca 28/1, office 1, Chisinau MD-2012, Republic of Moldova, Europe
Printed at: see last page
ISBN: 978-620-7-61574-2

THE CATGUT

RESULTS OF ITS IMPLEMENTATION IN PATIENTS WITH CHRONIC PELVIC INFLAMMATORY DISEASE.

LIZANDRA ESPINOSA CARÁS MIRTHA MARÍA PELÁEZ VEGA

2024

INTRODUCTION

In 1982, the Centers for Disease Control, following a symposium held in 1980 in Atlanta, USA, defined pelvic inflammatory disease (PID) as a clinical syndrome associated with the ascent of microorganisms from the vagina or cervix to the endometrium, fallopian tubes and contiguous structures, excluding those related to pregnancy, childbirth, puerperium and surgery (Erice, Román, Ulloa, Peláez, Juncal, 2008). The form of presentation can be acute or chronic. It is one of the most common pathologies affecting women of childbearing age. The impact of pelvic infection on a woman's physical condition ranges from asymptomatic or silent infection to increased morbidity, in some cases leading to death. It includes a variety of inflammatory conditions affecting the upper genital tract.Other factors that have been linked to an increase in PID include the use of intrauterine devices (IUDs), sexually transmitted, puerperal and post-abortion infections, and some surgical procedures, such as uterine dilatation and curettage, hysterosalpingography and a history of previous PID.It is estimated that by the year 2000, one in two women who reached reproductive age in the 1970s had an episode of pelvic inflammatory disease (P.I.D.), of whom 25% were hospitalised, 25% underwent major surgery and 20% were infertile. Between 8 - 20% of women with untreated gonococcal cervicitis and 8 - 10% of women with untreated chlamydial cervicitis were complicated by PID (Rigol 2004).PID is one of the most common infectious diseases in women of reproductive age. In the United States, it is estimated that more than 1 million women suffer an episode of acute pelvic inflammatory disease each year. No information is available on the prevalence and incidence of PID in the population of the Mexican Social Security Institute (IMSS). Nevertheless, we can say that PID is a health problem with a considerable cost. for society. In IMSS, PID is one of the main reasons for the demand for medical care in the population of sexually active women at the different levels of care as well as in the emergency services, so the therapeutic possibilities for this entity are still unlimited, Especially if we base ourselves on the concepts of Traditional Asian Medicine when we consider that energetic alterations in the Lower Jiao make it easier for pathogenic forms to settle in, causing processes of fullness, followed by chronic processes due to deficiencies in the channels linked to the female genital anatomy. As a consequence, dampness turns into phlegm, which turns into mucus that organises itself and affects the gynaecological structures in the first instance, causing chronic forms of the inflammatory and painful process. The origin of Traditional Chinese Medicine goes back beyond the dawn of history, it is a set of empirical methods, which are based on practical experience acquired over a long period of time. Not much is known about its origins, but it is strongly marked by three legendary figures, three mythical emperors (Borjas, Puig, 2002). The World Health Organisation (WHO) has been promoting the integrated use of traditional systems of medicine as part of primary health care programmes and has encouraged the study of their potential use as one of the basic pillars on which primary health care should be based (Authors' Collective, 2011). In Cuba, traditional medicine was practically unknown since the aboriginal population was almost entirely exterminated at the beginning of colonisation. The experiences of African ethnic groups and Spanish culture were incorporated into these scarce practices (Torres P, 2003). In 1991 Fidel directed the initiation of a programme for the rational use of medicinal plants, their scientific study and the generalisation of the resulting experiences as part of the programme of war preparation of the whole people, its practical implementation was expressed in 1993 by directive 8/93 of the Minister of the Revolutionary Armed Forces.(FAR). In 1995, Directive 26/95 of the Minister of the FAR and the 1st Programme for the Generalisation of Traditional and Natural Medicine (MTN) in the FAR were put into effect, and in 2001 the 2nd Programme for the Generalisation of MTN in the FAR was put into effect. In 2002, Agreement 4282 of the Executive Committee of the Council of Ministers was approved (MINFAR, 2010). In 2011, the Sixth Congress of the PCC approved guideline 158 of the Economic and Social Policy of the Party and the Revolution, which proposed paying attention to the development of Natural and Traditional Medicine.

Natural and traditional medicine is not an alternative method for the special period, but a discipline of the medical sciences that needs to be studied, perfected and maintained in the country. The application of these procedures for prevention, diagnosis and treatment is of great importance in peacetime, in contingency situations and in the preparation of the war of all the people, with its application we incorporate new therapeutic options to the medical services of the FAR (MINFAR, 2010).

Acupuncture (from the Latin acus: needle, puncture: to prick) is the name given to the Chinese therapeutic procedure Tshen-Ziu, which consists of the application of very fine needles to certain points on the skin (Álvarez, 1989).

Within the wide use of acupuncture therapy, gynaecological diseases in general and pelvic pain in particular, occupy a preferential place in terms of the effectiveness of the treatment, its harmlessness and the economy of medicinal resources. The creation of the Department of Traditional Asian Medicine made acupuncture treatment of pelvic pain possible, contributing to improving the combative disposition of women in our units (Reyes, Castro, Martínez, 2012).Catgut seeding therapy is a related technique of acupuncture by implanting small pieces of chrome-plated catgut inserted under certain parts of subcutaneous tissues for the treatment of diseases, the seeding sites, many of which with acupuncture points provide constant stimulation (usually 17-21 days). This type of treatment activates the physiological function and corrects the pathological condition of the body according to the purpose of curing diseases. In our province, its incidence is estimated at 60% of the female population of childbearing age. It is of great importance to know about this condition, as there is no programme in the world that supports it, which is why we consider it to be an aspect of priority attention for the training of health personnel.

In order to build a society aimed at the well-being, equity and equality of the people who make it up, their groups and communities need to acquire knowledge and skills, and the process of training plays an important role; this encompasses the educational processes aimed at improving or improving their human development.

The Guantanamo Military Region is not exempt from the impact that chronic pelvic inflammatory disease (CIPD) has on the physical condition of women and despite not constituting a prioritised programme, the incidence and prevalence, as well as the increase of this disease at an early age, obliges the doctor in the troops to seek solutions to deal with this health problem by incorporating habits into their behaviour that allow them to maintain a balance between health and disease, Therefore, we decided to conduct this research with the objective of evaluating the response to treatment with Catgut-therapy for chronic pelvic inflammatory disease in women in the Guantanamo Military Region in the period January - December 2023; Thus, we designed this study to respond to the following **scientific problem** statement:

Is the use of Traditional and Natural Medicine approaches effective in the treatment of this disease?

Purpose: Treatment scheme with the implantation of catgut in acupuncture points in patients with CIPD.

Based on the aforementioned object of the research, the **field of action** was established as the therapy with catgut implantation in acupuncture points as a technique related to acupuncture and a modality of traditional and natural medicine in the treatment of patients with CIPD.

With the result of the research, General Integral Medicine and Traditional and Natural Medicine in our Military Region will have another treatment modality for patients suffering from CIPD, which offers benefits to them and to the country, as well as the possibility of extending its application to other gynaecological pathologies and in this way achieving greater knowledge of this therapy among all professionals.

CHAPTER I

THEORETICAL FRAMEWORK- METHODOLOGICAL FRAMEWORK

THEORETICAL FRAMEWORK

Pelvic inflammatory disease (PID) consists of inflammation of the uterus (endometritis), fallopian tubes (salpingitis) and adjacent pelvic structures (tubulo-ovarian complex, pelvic peritonitis). PID causes significant medical, social and economic problems. Long-term sequelae, especially tubal factor infertility and extrauterine gestation, are frequent and very costly to treat. Medical treatment of PID should be immediate because sequelae are more frequent if treatment is delayed or inadequate (Alvarado, Chaguendo, 2008).

Pelvic inflammatory disease (PID) is an infection of the upper genital tract, including the different evolutionary phases of the infectious process, as well as the involvement of any of its locations, inflammation of the fallopian tubes being the most common form. This entity can appear at any time during a woman's reproductive life, but the risk of it appearing during adolescence and youth is much higher; it is accepted that in women under 20 years of age the risk is three times higher than in the 25-29 age group.

The higher frequency of this disease in adolescents and young people is explained, among other things, by the close association between sexually transmitted infections (STIs) and PID; it is now considered that a recent episode of STI is present in more than 90 % of all PID. As is widely known, the practice of risky sexual behaviours is a common characteristic in this age group, which makes this sector of the population at higher risk of STIs, PID and their sequelae (Peláez, 2012).

Multiple organisms have been implicated as aetiological agents of PID;

however, in most cases more than one organism is present. In different studies in the USA, 5-39% of women with a diagnosis of PID have been found with cervical and 0-10% with tubal PID, and serology has been found to be positive in 20-40% of women with a history of PID. As mentioned above, many Sometimes more than one micro-organism is involved; thus, a good group of them (anaerobes and aerobes) have been isolated from the upper third of the vagina in 25 to 30 % of women diagnosed with PID.

Although bacterial vaginosis is considered an endogenous infection, it is important to know that it has been found to be directly related to the genesis of polymicrobial PID. Thus, in women with severe PID, the germs involved in the pathogenesis of bacterial vaginosis are often found. Hence the importance of diagnosing and treating bacterial vaginosis, especially when scheduled gynaecological procedures are to be performed (Gutiérrez-Ramos, 2007).

The external genitalia should be examined for redness, fissures, ulcerations, warts and discharge. Inspection of the cervix is essential, as it may reveal mucopurulent endocervicitis or the presence of more than 10 polymorphonuclear leukocytes per microscopic field, which are of great magnitude when observed by Gram staining. During the bimanual pelvic examination, pain on mobilisation of the cervix and uterine adnexa is the cornerstone of the classic clinical diagnosis of PID, and its predictive value is 70 % when laparoscopic examination is performed as diagnostic confirmation.

Laboratory studies show that increased erythrocyte sedimentation rate, leukocytes and C-reactive protein are associated with PID. Ultrasonographic examination can show the presence of pelvic masses (tuboovarian abscesses), dilated tubes (pyosalpinx or hydrosalpinx) and fluid in the fundus of the pouch of Douglas. This is a non-invasive examination performed as an adjunct to the bimanual pelvic examination. Laparoscopic study was initially used for confirmation of the clinical diagnosis and is indicated in patients in whom, in addition to clinical suspicion of PID, the possibility of appendicitis, regional enteritis, extrauterine pregnancy, endometriosis, ovarian cyst, intra-abdominal bleeding due to ovulation or rupture of the corpus luteum is included. Laparoscopy also can be used for microbiological sampling. The most widely accepted explanation for the current increase in infertility is the impact of exogenous factors, due to the increase in sexually transmitted infections as a cause of PID, so that most cases of infertility can be attributed to tubal infections. Ectopic (tubal) pregnancy is also associated with previous PID and incomplete tubal lumen occlusion.

Women who have had PID are 6-10 times more likely to have an ectopic pregnancy. In most studies, about half of the tubes removed for ectopic pregnancy show signs of previous infection and patients report a history of PID. Another consequence known to all gynaecologists is chronic pelvic pain, defined as pain lasting 6 months or more, often related to the menstrual cycle and more pronounced during ovulation and the luteal phase; dyspareunia is common.

The proportion of patients with chronic pelvic pain increases with the number of episodes of PID and most have morphological changes of the uterine tubes and ovaries, related to the extension of pelvic, uterine and adnexal adhesions (Rigol, 2004). Factors that are important determinants in the development of acute salpingitis have now been clearly identified; sexually active adolescent girls are three times more at risk of developing pelvic inflammatory disease than sexually active women between 25 and 29 years of age. Adolescent girls are more susceptible to developing acute salpingitis because the endocervical columnar epithelium extends beyond the endocervix (called cervical ectopia), which produces a large area covered by columnar and squamocolumnar epithelium that is more susceptible to Chlamydia trachomatis infections. C. trachomatis does not appear to grow in the squamous cells of the exocervix and vagina. It has also been clearly identified that women who have numerous sexual partners are at increased risk of developing Acute Salpingitis (Pérez, 2007).

Bioenergetic and Natural Medicine, also called Traditional and Natural Medicine (TNM), known internationally as alternative, energetic and naturalistic or complementary, is part of the universal cultural heritage, i.e. concepts and practices that have been inherited from generation to generation. Its development has not been limited to the accumulation of knowledge derived from practice, but also to the design of a complete theoretical body, on the art of healing, integrated into modern health systems (Diaz, Lezcanol, Molerio, Hernández, 2001) (Collective of authors, 2009).

Natural and Bioenergetic Medicine is a branch of science based on the use of the wonders of nature and the body's energy to alleviate the patient's ailments. It includes a set of non-conventional methods, some of them recently developed from ancient techniques, with the aim of restoring and maintaining the harmonious functioning of the human organism (Acosta, García, Menéndez, Estrada, 2000).

We must have a proper use of lifestyle in patient care from the medical point of view, and when we are faced with a patient we must look at the patient as a whole and not only address the condition for which the patient comes to the consultation. To maintain proper mental and physical health there must be a biological balance. When this balance is broken, illness appears. In traditional Chinese medicine, this balance is called Yin and Yang, i.e. negative and positive, respectively, and in natural medicine it is a biopsychosocial balance.Health and illness are subjects of great universal interest, so it is necessary to work on the levels of prevention, treatment and rehabilitation that are possible with the chosen therapy, which also enables actions: analgesic, sedative and psychological, immunodefensive and homeostatic (Collective of authors, 2009). The Thesaurus of the US National Library of Medicine states that the therapies are considered complementary when used in addition to conventional treatments, and alternative when used instead of conventional treatment. The National Center for Complementary and Alternative Medicine (NCCAM) in the United States recognises 7 major areas of knowledge in the field of traditional medicine. They comprise:

Acupuncture, the practice of stimulating different points on the body (usually with needles) to heal; traditional oriental medicine, which deals with diagnosing energy disorders in the body; and homeopathy, which treats health problems with very diluted substances.

ro Phytotherapy or herbal medicine which includes the use of a wide range of plants used as medicine or for nutrition.

Manual healing that treats medical problems by manipulating and realigning various parts of the body. Perhaps the best known method is chiropractic, which focuses on the nervous system and the realignment of the spine. Other forms of manual healing include: massage; osteopathic medicine, which uses manipulation in addition to traditional medicine and surgical treatment; and contact healing, in which practitioners place their hands on or near the patient to direct energy to the diseased part of their body.

ro A diet that aims to introduce changes in a person's diet or lifestyle. Many people take supplemental nutrients if their usual diet does not contain enough vitamins or minerals, and people with chronic diseases such as heart disease or diabetes often change their diet or habits to keep the problem under control. This is one of the most useful forms of alternative care, because changing habits and diet not only helps treat numerous diseases, but can also prevent them. This part of alternative medicine is widely accepted for the western medical practitioner.

Mind and body control, which focuses on the role of the mind in disorders affecting the body. Hypnosis, a type of mindful sleep, can help some people deal with addictions, pain or anxiety, while treatments such as psychotherapy, meditation and yoga are used for relaxation.

Drugs and vaccines that have not yet been accepted by traditional medicine are also considered alternatives. Eventually, after much testing and FDA approval, some of these could become regularly prescribed treatments. ro Bioelectromagnetism, an emerging area of study that focuses on determining how changes in the body's electromagnetic fields can affect health, is based on the idea that electrical currents in all living organisms produce magnetic fields that extend beyond the body.

Traditional medicine in our country was brought to us in the 15th century by the Spaniards and later by Africans, Chinese and other cultures, but it mainly developed the use of medicinal plants, where the illustrious Dr. Juan Tomas Roig y Mesa, a pharmacist, stood out. There are verbal antecedents of the practice of traditional Chinese medicine in the city of Cárdenas in the province of Matanzas, where Dr. ChamBomBian worked, whose successes were remarkable in the decade before the end of the 19th century, especially in the prescription of medicinal plants. His work gave rise to the famous phrase: "not even a Chinese doctor can save him", with which he praised the high qualifications of the Asian doctor. However, it was not until 1980 that MINSAP established a plan for the development of Bioenergetic and Natural Medicine, although in 1991, the Commander-in-Chief decided to initiate a programme of known medicinal plants in the country, taking as an experience the return to the use of Natural Medicine that is taking place with increasing force in the countries of the world. industrialised. These guidelines were included in a programme of medicinal plants that formed part of the war preparation of all the people, and Directive 26/95 was implemented by the Minister of the FAR, for its execution not only including the National Health System but also other bodies and organisations, later replaced by Agreement 4282 of the Council of State. The National Thermalism Group was created with a multidisciplinary character that included medical professionals, engineers, geographers, architects and graduates in different specialities.

From this moment on, the Cuban National Health System developed a policy to expand the knowledge and use of TNM in close collaboration with the FAR, the MININT, the Cuban Academy of Sciences and other organisations. In our country, Traditional and Natural Medicine has been used since the arrival of the Chinese in Cuba, and experiences have been known since the war of the Mambises. With the triumph of the Revolution, this activity took off.

There are sufficient reasons to develop Traditional and Natural Medicine, due to the integral health-disease binomial, the doctor-patient relationship, the enrichment of therapeutic resources, the reduction of adverse reactions and the lower cost of its use (Hernández, Díaz, 2010).

In Cuba, Natural and Traditional Medicine (NTM) is not used as an additional or alternative procedure; rather, it is considered a true scientific discipline that can be applied by doctors or nurses, as it is relatively easy to learn.

The Cuban Ministry of Public Health laid the main foundations for action to improve the health levels of the Cuban population up to the year 2000. In this plan of objectives drawn up since 1992, the general guidelines also include the need to establish a programme for the accelerated introduction into the country of the main elements of alternative medicine, in particular the use of medicinal plants, acupuncture, as well as natural resources, mineral-medicinal waters and mud (Hernández, Díaz, 2010). Natural and Traditional Medicine today provides a service of high social value in Cuba, and is conceived as the incorporation of traditional knowledge from other peoples and the use of natural resources for the benefit of health. The new experiences that are emerging classify it as a speciality with a broad profile.

CHAPTER II
METHODOLOGICAL DESIGN OF THE STUDY

OBJECTIVE GENERAL

To evaluate treatment with catgut therapy in chronic pelvic inflammatory disease.

SPECIFIC OBJECTIVES

1. To characterise women with chronic pelvic inflammatory processes according to socio-demographic variables.
2. To determine the response to treatment with catgut therapy in women with chronic pelvic inflammatory processes.
3. Identify adverse reactions in the course of treatment.

METHODOLOGICAL DESIGN

A prospective descriptive longitudinal study was carried out in the Guantánamo Military Region, with the aim of evaluating the response to treatment with catgut-therapy for Chronic Pelvic Inflammatory Disease in the period January - December 2023. The research complied with the provisions of the Helsinki declaration, latest version corresponding to the Edinburgh Assembly, Scotland, October 2000. It was also governed by the state regulations in force in the Republic of Cuba for the performance of biological studies. This study was conducted in accordance with the principles of medical ethics and bioethics and international conventions to avoid harm; the confidentiality of the data collected and its exclusive use for scientific purposes was maintained. In compliance with the criteria of medical ethics, the objectives and importance of the research were explained to each patient included in the study, and informed consent was requested from them (appendix 1), where their willingness to participate and leave the study if they so wished was recorded, and prior coordination was carried out with the head of the military unit, political section, cadres, organisation and personnel and medical services (appendix 2).

The study universe consisted of 90 women and the sample consisted of only 42 women chosen by simple random sampling, who met the inclusion criteria and agreed to participate in the research.

Inclusion criteria

Women with untreated CIPD or with more than 5 days without specific topical or systemic treatment.

ro Agree to participate (Annex 1).

ro To be included in the Guantanamo Military Region.

Exclusion criteria.

ro Voluntary abandonment.

ro Patients affected by chronic decompensated systemic diseases.

❖ Exit criterion.

ro Move to another Military Region. ro Decide to abandon the research.

ro Progression of the disease.

ro Superimposed infection.

ro May he pass away.

Assessed by a first degree gynaecology specialist, the clinical and physical examination was considered for the diagnosis and definition of the patients to be included in the study.

The treatment schedule consisted of 21 days of catgut insertion, up to a total of 5 sessions, for a total duration of 15 weeks at the following acupuncture points:

► **Stomach 36 (ZUSANLI)**: Located in the anterior crural region, 3 cun below the DUBI point (E-35), a finger span lateral to the anterior border of the tibia. **Note:** The Point ZUSANLI is the HE-MAR point, the BEN-STATION point and the point representing the EARTH Movement of the Stomach channel. It is indicated in our study as a point that tonifies the general Qi (energy).

► **Vasoconception 4 (GUANYUAN or XIADANTIAN or XIAJI)**: It is located in the región hypogastric on the anterior midline 3 cun below the SHENQUE point (REN-8, in the centre of the navel) or 2 cun above the QUGU point (REN-2). It can warm and strengthen the original energy of Lower Sanyijiao, and also serves to strengthen the spleen and eliminate dampness. General tonification point. Frequent stimulation at this point is useful for strengthening health and resistance and for eliminating pathogenic factors·

Note: This point is the MU point of the Small Intestinal Canal. It is also the GUANYUAN is a JIAO HUI XUE (Meeting) point where the Renmai, Spleen, Liver and Kidney Channels meet. Due to the pathophysiological relationship that these channels have with the pathology under study, we considered including it in the selection of points for our treatment scheme.

► **Vasoconception 6 (QIHAI)**: Located in the hypogastric region, on the anterior midline 1.5 cun below the SHENQUE point (REN-8, navel centre). To regulate the circulation of the energy of the Vc meridian and that of the kidney, in order to eliminate dampness. It is considered a reservoir point of yang (Qi) and a gathering point for kidney energy. Tonifies the energy circuit.

► **Spleen 6 (SANYINJIAO)**: It is located in the posterior crural region, on the face of the spleen. posteromedial, 3 cun above the centre of the medial malleolus prominence, on the posteromedial border of the tibia

(Bilateral: 4 finger traverses 3 cun above the tip of the internal malleolus behind the internal border of the tibia, on the muscle mass).

It is the point of confluence of the 3 yin meridians of the foot which serve to strengthen the spleen, eliminate dampness and regulate liver and kidney functions. Homeostatic point recommended for genitourinary disorders of both sexes; menstrual disorders, disorders of the sexual sphere, chronic pelvic pain, pollakiuria, depression, physical and mental exhaustion. Point of dispersion, it disperses blood and energy (Xue and Qi), so that both circulate in balance; it harmonises the disagreement between Xue and Qi of the yin meridians.

Note: The SANYINJIAO Point is the GUAN or GROUP LUO point at which the three

Leg YIN channels Liver, Spleen and Kidney.

► **Liver 2 (XINGJIAN):** It is located on the dorsum of the foot, in the depression anterior to the firstmetatatarsophalangeal joint, at 0.5 cun behind the interdigital border of the two first toes. **Note**: This is the YING-MANTIAL point, the BEN DE point.

DISPERSION and the point representing the FIRE Movement of the Liver channel.

► **Stomach 40 (FENGLONG):** It is located over the anterior crural region, 8 cun below the **stomach.** from the DUBI point (E-35), on the lateral border of the tibialis anterior muscle. **Note:** The FENGLONG point is the LUO-LINK point of the Stomach channel. Also known as the PASSAGE point, it connects the Stomach and Spleen channels.

Lumbar puncture trocars No.18 and 20 were used, the tip of which is slightly tapered (thus widening the bevel), flattening the end of the anterior part of the needle which is slightly longer than the needle tube, a chrome-plated Catgut thread for medical use No. 0.3 and 0.4 was selected.

According to what we used, the Catgut thread was cut into small pieces that fluctuated between 0.5 and 1 cm in length. With an "X" we marked with the pressure of the fingernail of the hand with previous sterilisation of the local skin, the thread was placed in the cavity of the needle in its anterior part, and the needle was quickly inserted into the skin up to 1.5 cm deep. The needle should not be left in the adipose tissue as it is more difficult to absorb, the trocar was pulled back slightly (0.5 cm) and the needle itself was pushed into the trocar to push the Catgut out of the trocar tube, thus implanting the Catgut thread into the tissue.

With the needle withdrawn about 1 cm below the skin, the Catgut fibre was completely pushed out of the trocar and the needle was removed. In case of bleeding, pressure was applied for a while with sterile cotton or swab. There were 21-day cycles for each implant. The implantation was done in 5 sessions.

The patients underwent a first follow-up consultation at the second session after the start of treatment and a follow-up consultation at the end of the treatment (week 5) in which the evolution was evaluated:

Good: when more than 90 % of the symptoms have disappeared.

Regular: when between 60 and 89 % disappeared.

Poor: when symptom resolution was less than 59%.

Adverse reactions were classified according to the degree of intensity according to the conventional classification:

1. Mild: when the adverse reaction does not significantly interfere with the subject's normal functioning.

ro This may be a transitory event.

It may be a non-treatable event.

2. Moderate: when the adverse reaction causes impairment of the subject's normal functioning without constituting a health risk, it may be

an event that requires treatment and yields to treatment.

3. Severe: when the adverse reaction causes significant impairment of the subject's normal functioning, function or organ structure without being life-threatening.

It may be an event of minor clinical significance that prolongs that present in its most severe form.

ro It may be an event that requires treatment and does not yield to treatment.
ro This may be an event involving temporary interruption of treatment.
4. Serious: an adverse event leading to death or reduced life expectancy of the subject.

It may lead to definitive discontinuation of treatment.

ro It may be an event requiring emergency medical or surgical intervention to eliminate or prevent impairment of function or permanent damage to an organ structure.

A serious adverse reaction is any untoward medical occurrence at any dose and in addition to the above:

ro Requires hospitalisation or prolongation of an existing hospitalisation.
It results in significant or persistent incapacity, disability or invalidity, where disability is defined as any substantial interruption of the ability to carry out vital functions.

ro Produces a birth defect or congenital anomaly.
It does not include an adverse reaction which, if it occurred in a more severe form, could have caused death.

5. Unexpected adverse reaction: an unexpected adverse reaction is one whose severity is inconsistent with the product information so far available (information contained in the package leaflet or package insert

for an approved product and contained in t h e investigator's brochure or protocol).

Example:

ro Adverse reaction not previously described.

ro Adverse reaction previously described in the available literature, but o c c u r r i n g with increased frequency, increased pathological severity or progression, or a more precise description.

TECHNIQUES AND PROCEDURES:

Obtaining the information: An exhaustive bibliographical review was carried out in accordance with the chosen topic and depending on the proposed objectives, in the Provincial Library, the library of the General Hospital of Guantánamo, the library of the University of Medical Sciences of Santiago and Guantánamo, among others. In addition, using new techniques for obtaining information, searches were carried out in virtual medical libraries in our country and abroad. The information and research was collected through consultations carried out by the authors.

Processing and analysis of the information: It was processed on a Pentium V computer using simple tables and double-entry association, distribution and frequency tables, as well as graphs used as a unit of summary, numbers to the tenth decimal place and percentages in correspondence to the total population attended with the diagnosis under study. The source of all the tables used was the consultation and clinical history, by the method of analysis and synthesis, induction and deduction, historical and logical in its descriptive variant.

CHAPTER III
ANALYSIS AND DISCUSSION OF RESULTS

ANALYSIS AND DISCUSSION OF THE RESULTS

Regardless of the empiricism that characterised our practice in its beginnings, the results achieved demonstrated the ample possibilities of improving the quality of life of our women in the troops, in spite of being an investigation that does not reach a full and absolute application of traditional medicine, as we did not take into account essential aspects such as the traditional Chinese diagnosis in each selected patient; as a guide for therapeutic actions, in function of re-establishing the energy balance of the patients; an implicit objective to achieve in a second stage of this work. As you will be able to analyse, in all cases we directed our therapeutics to treatments with techniques that acted from the outside. Nevertheless, the results obtained are positive.It is important to note that the insufficient literature available on this subject made it impossible for us to discuss and compare our findings with those of other authors; However, our reasoning regarding pain, leucorrhoea and associated symptoms, summarised in the clinical evolution and response to treatment, allows us to affirm that the sustained action of chrome catgut on biologically active points not only regulates the bioenergetic balance (yin-yan) of the organism, but also the energy (Qi), blood (Xue), body fluids (jin ye) and damaged meridians, thus fulfilling the golden rule of acupuncture therapeutics: Treat the affected meridian (Vc), a meridian of nearby circulation (Bp) and a point at a distance (E 36 and E 40).

Table 1: Relationship between age group and marital status of patients with chronic pelvic inflammatory disease. Catgut implantation in patients with chronic pelvic inflammatory disease.

Age groups (Years)	Marital status									
	Singles		Married		Campaigns		Widows		Total	
	No	%	No	%	No	%	No	%	No	%
20- 24	9	21.4	0	0	2	4.8	0	0	11	26.2
25-29	3	7.1	5	12.0	7	16.6	0	0	15	35.8
30-34	0	0	1	2.4	3	7.1	0	0	4	9.5
35-39	1	2.4	2	4.8	4	9.5	0	0	7	16.6
40-44	0	0	1	2.4	3	7.1	0	0	4	9.5
45-49	0	0	0	0	1	2.4	0	0	1	2.4
Total	13	30.9	9	21.6	20	47.5	0	0	42	100

As can be seen in table 1, women aged 25 to 29 years predominate with 15 patients (35.8 %), followed by 11 women aged 20 to 24 years (26.2 %), then 7 women (25.8 %), followed by 11 women aged 20 to 24 years (26.2 %).35 to 39 years old (16.6%), followed by the age groups 30 to 34 and 40 to 44 years old with 4 females (9.5%) and 4 females (9.5%). %), only 1 woman aged 45-49 years, representing 2.4 % of the total study population. In terms of marital status, 20 women (47.5 %) were married, followed by 13 single (30.9 %), then 9 married (21.6 %), and no widows were found in our study.In terms of marital status, single women prevailed with 13 (30.9%), including 9 patients aged 20 to 24 years (21.4%), then 3 women aged 25 to 29 years (7.1%), followed by the 35 to 39 age group with only 1 female (2.4%) of the total population. Of the married women, 5 were aged 25 to 29 years (12.0 %), 2 were aged 35 to 39 years (4.8 %), followed by the age groups 30 to 34 and 40 (4.8 %). to 44 years with 1 female each (2.4% of the total). Accompanied women was the marital status with the highest number of patients, with a total of 20 women, in the 25-29 age group with 7 women (16.6 % of the total). %), 4 women aged 35-39 (9.5 %), 3 women in the age groups 30-34 and 40-44 representing 7.1 % of the total study population, followed by 2 and 1 women aged 20-24 and 45-49 with 4.8 and 2.4 % respectively. According to Reyes A, Castro J, Martínez G, in their study: "Tratamiento de las algias pélvicas con acupuntura" (Treatment of pelvic pain with acupuncture), the ages at which pelvic pain most frequently manifested were those between 15 and 25 and 26 and 35 years of age, with 27.28 and 32.29 % respectively, age groups that correspond to the fullest oestrogenic period and the greatest sexual activity of women, coincidentally our study yielded similar results.Other authors, such as Dr. Jorge Peláez Mendoza, in his study "EIP y adolescencia", state that this entity can appear at any time during a woman's reproductive life, but the risk of it appearing during adolescence is much higher; it is accepted that in women under 20 years of age, the risk is 3 times higher than in the 25-29 age group, considering EIP to be the most frequent serious infection in women between 16 and 25 years of age.In reviews we have also found that authors such as Dr. Juan Pablo Alvarado Forero Professor of Gynaecology & Obstetrics at the University of Cauca and Dr. José Enrique Chaguendo García Professor of Gynaecology & Obstetrics at the University of Cauca, state that in Colombia, sexually transmitted diseases, alone or with PCIDs as their sequelae, are one of the leading causes of gynaecological consultations and are among the first ten causes of morbidity in the economically active population. It is the leading cause of acute lower abdominal pain. It is estimated that there are 3 to 9 cases per 1000 women aged 15 to 44 years and 12 to 18 cases per 1000 women aged 15 to 24 years per year. In her study "Utility of Acupunctural Therapy in Patients with Pelvic Inflammation",

Berna Benita Pérez Sánchez states that in the United States of America it is estimated that every year more than one million women are treated for acute salpingitis (AS). The incidence is highest in adolescents and women under the age of 25. This condition and its complications are the cause of more than 2.5 million consultations and more than 150,000 surgical procedures each year.

18-20 out of every 1000 women aged 15-24 years acquire salpingitis each year, with HS being the cause of 5-20% of hospitalisations in gynaecology departments in the USA. Eight to 20 % of untreated women with endocervical infection by Neisseria gonorrhoeae or Chlamydia trachomatis develop acute salpingitis; more than 25 % of patients with acute salpingitis are under 25 years of age and 75 % are nulliparous. Acute Salpingitis is responsible for approximately 20% of infertility cases (Perez, 2007).Simultaneously our study agrees with these results as it shows the highest number of 15 to 11 women aged 25 to 29 and 20 to 24 representing 35.7% and 26.2% respectively of the sample taken. The lowest figure was 1 woman aged 45-49 years, representing 35.7% and 26.2% respectively of the sample taken.2.4 % of the study population, considering that PID is more frequent in young women. In our opinion as authors we confirm with our work that Pelvic Inflammatory Disease (PID) is a frequent disease in young women between 20 and 30 years old, sexually active adolescents are more susceptible to develop this pathology, as risk factors are a history of previous episodes of Pelvic Inflammatory Disease, or sexually transmitted disease (STD), recent insertion of Intra Uterine Device, sexual partner with urethritis or asymptomatic sexually transmitted disease.

Table 2: Relationship between age groups and schooling of patients with chronic pelvic inflammatory disease.

Age groups (Years)	Schooling									
	Primary		Secondary		Baccalaureate		University		Total	
	No	%	No	%	No	%	No	%	No	%
20- 24	0	0	0	0	9	21.4	2	4.8	11	26.2
25-29	0	0	0	0	5	12.0	10	23.8	15	35.8
30-34	0	0	0	0	1	2.4	3	7.1	4	9.5
35-39	0	0	0	0	0	0	7	16.6	7	16.6
40-44	0	0	0	0	0	0	4	9.5	4	9.5
45-49	0	0	0	0	0	0	1	2.4	1	2.4
Total	0	0	0	0	15	35.8	27	64.2	42	100

When analysing table 2 for discussion, we can see that women between 25 and 29 years of age predominate with 15 patients (35.7%), followed by 11 women between 20 and 24 years of age (26.2%), then 7 women between 35 and 39 years (16.6%), followed by women between 30 and 39 years of age (16.6%).34 and 40-44 years old with 4 females (9.5 %), only 1 lady aged 45-49 years old representing 2.4 % of the total study population.In terms of level of education, 27 women (64.2 %) were university graduates, followed by 15 women with a baccalaureate (35.8 %). Among the university students, 10 women (23.8 %) were aged 25 to 29, followed by 9 women aged 20 to 24 (21.4 %) with a bachelor's degree, then 7 university students (16.6 %) in the 35 to 39 age group, 5 in the 25 to 29 age group (12.0 %), 4 university students (9.5 %) in the 40 to 44 age group, 3 university students in the 30 to 40 age group (9.5 %), 3 women in the 30 to 40 age group (9.5 %), 3 women with a bachelor's degree in the 25 to 29 age group (12.0 %), 4 university students in the 35 to 39 age group (9.5 %), and 3 women in the 30 to 40 age group (9.5 %).34 years old (7.1 %), 2 university students aged 20-24 (4.8 %) and 1 each from the age groups 30-34 and 45-49 (2.4 %) from high school and university respectively.Regardless of the fact that it has not been found in the consulted bibliography and reviewsIn the case of the ICPS, the results of the survey were analysed and compared with those described above, in order to ascertain the behaviour of the ICPS in relation to the schooling variable,We can say that university students stood out with 27 women (64.2 %) of the total population under study, which allowed us to perceive that the educational level does not influence the suffering of CIPD and that all women, regardless of their schooling, are exposed to suffer from CIPD.In our opinion as authors, we consider that no woman of childbearing age, young and sexually active is free from suffering from PCID, as cultural and educational level does not save us from suffering from episodes of this entity.

Table 3: Symptoms present in patients with chronic pelvic inflammatory disease.

SymptomsStart of TTOEnd of TTO

	NO.	%	NO.	%
Lower abdominal pain	42	100	13	31,1
Leucorrhoea	11	26,9	6	14,3
Fever	-	-	-	-
Dyspareunia	38	90,4	6	14,3
Gastrointestinal symptoms	-	-	-	-

On examining the results shown in this table for analysis and discussion, we can see that the main symptoms present in the patients at the beginning and end of the treatment are shown. We noticed that initially lower abdominal pain predominated in the 42 women in question (100

%), followed by 38 women (90.4 %) with dyspareunia, only 11 had leucorrhoea (26.9 %), and none had fever or gastrointestinal symptoms.At the end of treatment 13 patients remained with lower abdominal pain, representing 31.1%, 6 with leucorrhoea and dyspareunia (14.3%), symptoms which, although not measurable in the table from a qualitative point of view, were clearly present, but they underwent changes in the intensity and frequency of their occurrence; they were also related to the results achieved in the response to treatment.The collective of Mexican authors in their study "Diagnosis and treatment of PID in sexually active women over 14 years of age" state that in a cohort study it was shown that the most common symptoms were:

ro Abdominal pain for 90%.

ro Leucorrhoea for 70%.

ro Irregular bleeding for 40%.

ro 30 % of the patients had a history of Intra Uterine Device (IUD) (Authors' Collective, 2009).

In the Revista Cubana de Obstetricia y Ginecología in 2010, doctors Daisy Hernández Durán and Orlando Díaz Mitjans state in their article that pelvic inflammatory disease can present with the following symptoms:

Lower abdominal pain (including adnexal pain, dyspareunia). It is the most common symptom

95 % of the cases are frequent.

Increased vaginal discharge, 74% abnormal discharge.

ro Abnormal bleeding (intermenstrual, post-coital) in 45%.

ro Urinary symptoms in 35%.

ro Vomiting in 14 %.

They also argue that the absence of symptoms is possible (Hernández, Díaz Mitjans 2010).

PID often presents with few or no signs or symptoms. Pain is the most frequent symptom, of variable intensity in relation to the extent and severity of the process; it increases with changes in position and with ambulation, becomes intolerable when PID extends to the peritoneum, and forces the patient to remain lying down.

Fever may rise to 39 or 40 ^{o}C and is accompanied by chills. Leucorrhoea often precedes the onset of pelvic pain by 10-20 days. Approximately ¾ of all women report increased vaginal discharge. Gastrointestinal symptoms are rare in mild to moderate PID (Rigol, 2004). In the opinion of the authors, we believe with our work that Pelvic Inflammatory Disease (PID) is an entity in which it is common for young women to develop this pathology frequently, reporting to the doctors in the military units a history of previous episodes of Pelvic Inflammatory Disease or recent insertion of Intra Uterine Device accompanied by lower abdominal pain in almost 100% of them, related to leucorrhoea and dyspareunia among other symptoms. Therefore, we agree with the criteria originally set out by the authors cited above.

Table 4: Assessment of treatment response in patients with chronic pelvic inflammatory disease.

Age groups (Years)	RESPONSE TO TREATMENT						TOTAL	
	GOOD		REGULAR		MALA			
	No.	%	No.	%	No.	%	No.	%
20- 24	8	19.0	2	4.8	1	2.4	11	26.2
25-29	7	16.6	5	12.0	3	7.1	15	35.8
30-34	3	7.1	1	2.4	-	-	4	9.5
35-39	3	7.1	3	7.1	1	2.4	7	16.6
40-44	2	4.8	1	2.4	1	2.4	4	9.5
45-49	-	-	1	2.4	-	-	1	2.4
Total	23	54.6	13	31.1	6	14.3	42	100

In examining the results set out in the current table for analysis and discussion, the following results are presented in the following table we can assess that women between 25 and 29 years of age predominate with 15 patients (35.8 %).%), followed by 11 women aged 20-24 (26.2 %), then 7 women aged 35-39 (16.6 %), followed by the age groups 30-34 and 40-44 years with 4 females (9.5 %), only 1 female aged 45-49 years representing 2.4 % of the total study population.

RESPONSES TO TREATMENT

Good:

The age group 20 to 24 years old predominated with 8 females (19.0 %), followed by 25 to 29 years old with 7 females (19.0 %), followed by 25 to 29 years old with 7 females (19.0 %). women (16.6 %), then the age groups 30-34 and 35-39 with 3 women (7.1 %), followed by the age group 40-44 with 2 women (4.8 %).

Regular:

The age group 25 to 29 years predominated with 5 females (12.0 %), followed by 35 to 39 years with 3 females (7.1 %), then the age group 20 to 24 years with 2 females (4.8 %), followed by the age groups 30 to 34, 40 to 44 and 45 to 49 years with 1 female (2.4 %).

Mala:

The age group 25-29 years predominated with 3 females (7.1 %), followed by the age groups 20-24, 35-39 and 40-44 with 1 female (2.4 %).In their research "Sowing Catgut in acupuncture points as a treatment for symptomatic uterine fibroids", doctors Díaz M. and Berdión B. from the Higher Institute of Medical Sciences, Faculty of Medicine No. 1. Faculty of Medicine No. 1. Santiago de Cuba, it can be seen that as the acupuncture treatment was applied, the patients in the study group gradually eliminated the symptom or evolved favourably with respect to their pain intensity; however, in the sixth therapeutic session, even 74.3% of those who received medication to improve their clinical picture continued to be symptomatic to a greater or lesser degree.

Associated with the fibroma, leucorrhoea was present in 31.4 and 25.7 % of the patients in the first and second groups, in that order; by the third treatment session, this sign had been eradicated in all those treated with catgut, but not in 11.4 % of the controls; by the sixth treatment session, the latter were also free of this bothersome manifestation.

Genital bleeding affected 71.4 % of the women in the 2 groups at the start of treatment, respectively; by the sixth session, it was completely controlled in the women in the 2 groups. The treatment given by catgut sowing on acupuncture points was effective in patients with symptomatic uterine fibroids, as the clinical manifestations of pain, bleeding, bleeding and light pain disappeared in 65.7 % of patients with symptomatic fibroids. The treatment given by sowing catgut on acupuncture points was effective in patients with symptomatic uterine fibroids, since the clinical manifestations consisting of pain, bleeding, leucorrhoea and other associated symptoms disappeared in almost all of them (94.3 %), in addition to having proved to be comparatively superior to the conventional therapy. By the third treatment session, most of the members of the study group had experienced a significant improvement in the symptoms and signs of the condition, and by the sixth session, more than three quarters of those treated with the oriental technique were asymptomatic; in the controls, on the other hand, only 5.7 % of the controls showed total improvement, with a predominance of those who continued without any change in their clinical picture (Díaz, Berdión, 2000).In the opinion of the authors, we consider that our results open up a greater perspective in relation to the treatment of women suffering from CIPD, since the improvement of symptoms could mean hope for the possible recovery of these patients and their incorporation into the troops, which is why we consider that natural and traditional medicine, particularly acupuncture with its variant: catgut sowing, should be incorporated into the therapy of gynaecological disorders and the use of this procedure should become generalised.

Table 5: Adverse reactions to treatment in patients with chronic pelvic inflammatory disease.

Adverse reactions	Treatment sessions										Total	
	1st		2nd		3rd		4th		5th			
	No.	%	No.	%	No	%	No	%	No.	%	No.	%
Slight	5	12	3	7,1	1	2,4	-	-	-	-	9	21,4
Moderate	-	-	-	-	-	-	-	-	-	-	-	-
Severe	-	-	-	-	-	-	-	-	-	-	-	-
Serious	-	-	-	-	-	-	-	-	-	-	-	-
Reaction unexpected adverse	-	-	-	-	-	-	-	-	-	-	-	-

Table 5, which shows the adverse reactions associated with the treatment sessions in patients with chronic pelvic inflammatory disease, shows that the adverse reactions present were slight, being pain and local reddening at the level of the applied tools, a total of 9 women (21.4 %), in the first treatment session only 5 patients (12.0 %), and in the second session only 5 patients (12.0 %) were affected. %), the second 3 women (7.1 %) and the third only 1 female (2.4 %). Although we did not find any bibliography for comparison, in our opinion as the author, we consider that acupuncture therapy with catgut therapy is favourable for women with gynaecological conditions, since, as can be seen, they evolve favourably with respect to the intensity of the symptoms, and the adverse reactions are minimal, with a favourable clinical evolution. As can be seen, almost all the women included in the study group achieved total improvement. In the first session, 5 women were described as having only However, by the fifth treatment session, no adverse effects were reported and most of the symptoms were eradicated.

CONCLUSIONS

In the clinical epidemiological characterisation, the predominant age groups were women aged 20-24 and 25-29, accompanied and with a university education. The majority of the patients evolved favourably with the applied therapy; the catgut implantation had a positive influence on the relief and disappearance of symptoms and other discomforts that had an unfavourable impact on their well-being and led to a reduction in the demand for medical services due to the affectation of the combative disposition. There was no increase in expected adverse reactions in general and no serious and unexpected events were identified in the course of treatment.

RECOMMENDATIONS

Generalise this therapeutic modality in all institutions of the Medical Services of the FAR, where this condition constitutes a health problem, propose a common research protocol for its application in order to implement strategies that facilitate its development.ro Continue to deepen the design of clinical-therapeutic research in this area and include traditional Chinese diagnosis as a guide for therapeutic actions, in order to restore the energy balance of patients.ro Evaluate the cost-benefit of this procedure for its possible inclusion in therapeutic guidelines because it is effective, and above all because of the low percentage of adverse reactions.ro In short, to establish a Traditional Medicine Service that works together and in harmony with Western Medicine, achieving a high level of wellbeing for patients in our health areas.

REFERENCES

Acosta M., García R., Menéndez S., Estrada C. (2000). Application of oleozon as an alternative medicine in nursing. Therapeutic and economic results. 3rd International Congress on ozone applications, Havana. Book of abstracts, 30,

Alvarado J, Chaguendo J (2008). Clinical guidelines for the care of pelvic inflammatory disease (PID).

Álvarez TA (1989). Manual de acupuntura. Havana City: Editorial Ciencias Médicas.

Ozone applications. Rev CENIC Cienc. Chem. (1989): 20 (1, 2, 3) 81.

Baracaldo N, Morell L and Baracaldo A. (2014). Treatment of vaginal sepsis with homeopathy.

Bocci V, Luzzy. Corradeschi F., Paulesu Ld., Stefan A. (1993) Studies on the biological effects of ozone. Lymphokine cytokine ress: 12 - 121.

Bocci V. Ozonetherapy today. (1995) Proc. 12th Ozone World Congress, Lille, France, Vol. Ozone in Medicine. 13 - 27.

Borjas D, Puig R. (2002). Basic Elements of Bioenergetic Medicine for students of Medical Sciences. Havana: Editorial Ciencias Médicas.

Authors' collective (2009) Diagnosis and treatment of pelvic inflammatory disease in sexually active women over 14 years of age. Mexico: Ministry of Health.

Collective of authors (2011). Methodology for the work of Natural and Traditional Medicine.

Ministry of Public Health. Havana.

Daniel R, Moya S. (1992) Dermatophytes isolated from the interdigital spaces of the feet without clinical lesions. Rev cubana medmilit; 21(1):50.

Ozone Research Centre. (1996) Experiences of a decade of work in

Cuba: perspectives. Havana city.

Diaz M., Lezcanol. Molerio J. And Hernández F. (2001). "Spectroscopic characterization of ozonides with biological activity", ozone sci. & eng., 23(1):35 - 40

Díaz M. Floirán and Berdión B. (2000) Catgut sowing in acupuncture points as a treatment for symptomatic uterine fibroids. Higher Institute of Medical Sciences. Faculty of Medicine No. 1. Santiago de Cuba, Cuba. Approved: January 12, (Cited: 2015 Jan 23).

Erice A I, Román L, Ulloa V, Peláez J, Juncal (2008). In: Álvarez R. Medicina General Integral.

Falcón I., Menéndez, S., Simón R. D. (2000) Solution for Epidermophytosis of the feet in members of the FAR. Rev. Cubana Med. Militar; 29 (2): 98-102.

Falcón I. Menéndez, S. Simón R. D. (2002). Efficacy of oleozon in the treatment of epidermophytosis. Mycoses, 45(8):329 - 333,

Gutiérrez-Ramos M. (2007) Pelvic inflammatory disease: etiopathogenesis. Rev Per Gynecol Obstet [internet]. 53: 228-233.

Hernández D, Díaz O. (2010) Pelvic inflammatory disease. Rev. Cub Obstetrics and Gynaecology [internet]. 36(4): 613-631.

Hernández D, Díaz O. (2010) The use of ozone in medicine. 2nd rev ed Hang pub:7-100.

Pérez B. (2007) Utility of acupuncture therapy in patients with pelvic inflammation Havana City.

MINFAR (2010). Guía de procedes terapéuticos de la Medicina Natural y Tradicional en las FAR. Atención Médica Básica. Ciudad de la Habana.

Morris, G. Menéndez, S. et al. Ozone treatment in gynaecology. First Ibero-Latin American congress on ozone applications. Cnic - CIMEQ, 31 October 1990.

Reyes A, Castro J, Martínez G. (2012) Treatment of pelvic algia with acupuncture. Rev. Virt Medic Tradicional China [internet].

Rigol O (2004) Obstetricia y Ginecología. Havana City: Editorial Ciencias Médicas.

Pryor A. and Rice R. G. (1998) Introduction to the use of the ozone in food processing applications.

Ozone news, 26 - 28.

Peláez M. (2012) Pelvic inflammatory disease and adolescence. Rev Cub Ginecol Obstet Torres P. (2003). Nursing in Natural and Traditional Medicine. Havana: Editorial Ciencias

Medical;

Stein, J.H. (1987) Internal Medicine. Volume II. Vol. I. Ed. Revolucionaria. Havana. P 1429.

ANNEXES

Annex 1. Informed Consent

Our work is an investigation into chronic pelvic inflammatory disease in women in the Guantánamo Military Region treated with MNT, which will allow us to improve the conduct to be followed in the FAR before this pathology.

Your participation is anonymous, we will respect your opinion and the results of the survey will only be used for scientific purposes. We appreciate the help you can give us, we ask for your understanding. You are free to leave the research if you wish or not to participate in it.

If you agree, we count on your approval. By signing I am of sound mind.

Signature of the Patient

Name and surname:

Age:

Marital status:

✓ Single:

✓ Married:

✓ Accompanied:

✓ Divorced:

✓ Widow:

Schooling:

✓ Primary:

✓ Secondary:

✓ Pre-university:

✓ University:

Response to treatment:

✓ Good:

✓ Regular:

✓ Mala:

Adverse reactions:

✓ Lightweight:

✓ Moderate:

✓ Severe:

✓ Serious:

√ Unexpected:

Symptoms present:

√ Lower abdominal pain:

√ Leucorrhoea:

√ Fever:

√ Dyspareunia or coitalgia:

√ Gastrointestinal symptoms:

Annex 4. Pictures of catgut

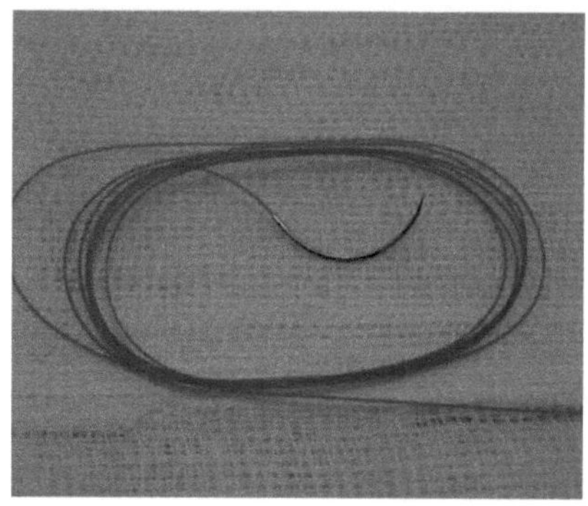

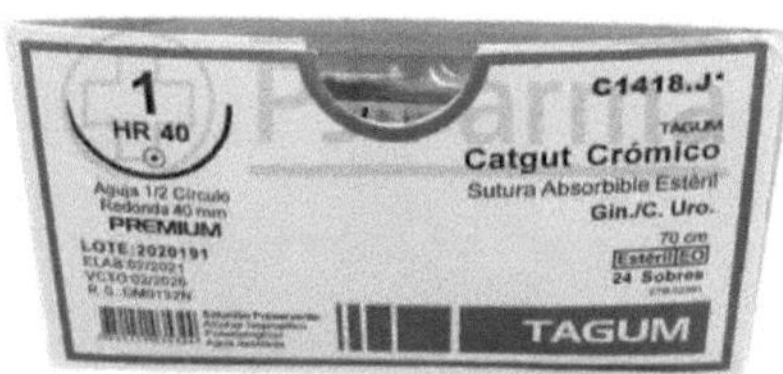

CONTENTS

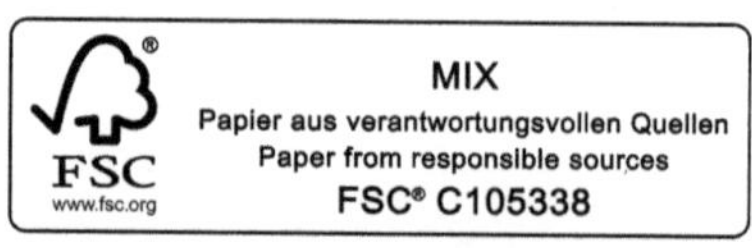

Printed by Books on Demand GmbH, Norderstedt / Germany